# THYRO

## BOLSTER RECIPES

### 14-DAY MEAL PLAN

### PLUS 300 DAYS RECIPES

MICHELLE CARSON

# CONTENT

# CHAPTER ONE: understanding thyroid health

## What is Thyroid

The thyroid is a small butterfly-shaped gland located in the front of the neck, just below Adam's apple. It is a part of the endocrine system, which is responsible for producing and regulating hormones in the body. The thyroid gland plays a crucial role in regulating various metabolic processes and controlling the body's energy levels.

The thyroid produces two primary hormones: thyroxine (T4) and triiodothyronine (T3). These hormones are involved in regulating metabolism, growth, and development, as well as influencing the functioning of almost every organ in the body. The production and release of thyroid hormones are controlled by the pituitary gland, which produces thyroid-stimulating hormone (TSH). TSH prompts the thyroid gland to produce and release T4 and T3.

Thyroid disorders can occur when the thyroid gland produces either too much or too little thyroid hormone. Common thyroid conditions include hypothyroidism (an underactive thyroid), hyperthyroidism (an overactive thyroid), and thyroid nodules. Symptoms of thyroid disorders can vary but often include fatigue, weight changes, mood swings, hair loss, changes in heart rate, and difficulty regulating body temperature.

Diagnosis of thyroid disorders typically involves blood tests to measure hormone levels and imaging tests, such as ultrasounds or scans, to evaluate the structure of the thyroid gland. Treatment options vary depending on the specific thyroid condition but may include medication, radioactive iodine therapy, surgery, or lifestyle changes. It's important to consult a healthcare professional for proper diagnosis and management of thyroid disorders.

## How Does Thyroid works

The thyroid gland, located in the neck, produces hormones called thyroxine (T4) and triiodothyronine (T3) that play a crucial role in regulating metabolism and various body functions. Here's a summary of how the thyroid works:

1. The hypothalamus, a region in the brain, detects low levels of thyroid hormones and releases thyrotropin-releasing hormone (TRH).
2. TRH signals the pituitary gland, located at the base of the brain, to release thyroid-stimulating hormone (TSH).
3. TSH travels to the thyroid gland and stimulates it to produce and release T4 and a smaller amount of T3 into the bloodstream.
4. T4 is converted to T3 in various tissues throughout the body, and both T3 and T4 bind to specific receptors within cells.
5. T3 and T4 regulate metabolism, energy production, growth, and development by influencing gene expression and cellular processes.
6. As T3 and T4 levels increase, they provide negative feedback to the hypothalamus and

pituitary gland, reducing the release of TRH and TSH, respectively.

7. This negative feedback loop helps maintain a stable balance of thyroid hormones in the body.

Thyroid disorders can occur when there is an imbalance in the production or regulation of thyroid hormones. Hypothyroidism results from insufficient hormone production, leading to a slower metabolism, fatigue, and weight gain. Hyperthyroidism occurs when there is excessive hormone production, causing a faster metabolism, weight loss, and increased heart rate.

Proper diagnosis and management of thyroid disorders are important for maintaining overall health and well-being. Treatment options may include hormone replacement therapy, medications, radioactive iodine therapy, or surgery, depending on the specific condition. Regular monitoring and working with healthcare professionals are essential for optimal thyroid health.

## Signs Of Thyroid Disorder

Thyroid disorders can present with various signs and symptoms. Here are some common signs that may indicate a thyroid disorder:

1. Fatigue and weakness: Feeling excessively tired or weak, even after getting adequate rest, can be a symptom of both hypothyroidism and hyperthyroidism.

2. Weight changes: Unexplained weight gain or difficulty losing weight despite efforts can be associated with hypothyroidism. Conversely, sudden weight loss or an increased appetite can be signs of hyperthyroidism.

3. Changes in heart rate: Hypothyroidism can cause a slower heart rate (bradycardia), while hyperthyroidism can lead to a faster heart rate (tachycardia) or palpitations.

4. Mood changes: Depression, irritability, anxiety, and mood swings can be symptoms of both hypothyroidism and hyperthyroidism.

5. Intolerance to cold or heat: Feeling excessively cold or having an increased sensitivity to cold temperatures is often associated with hypothyroidism. On the other hand, feeling hot, sweating excessively, or having an increased sensitivity to heat can be signs of hyperthyroidism.

6. Changes in bowel habits: Constipation is a common symptom of hypothyroidism, while hyperthyroidism can cause more frequent bowel movements or diarrhea.

7. Changes in menstrual cycle: Women with thyroid disorders may experience irregular or heavier menstrual periods.

8. Changes in hair, skin, and nails: Dry skin, brittle nails, and hair loss (including thinning of the eyebrows) can occur with hypothyroidism.

Hyperthyroidism may cause thinning hair and fragile nails.

9. Muscle aches and weakness: Muscle pain, stiffness, weakness, or cramps can be symptoms of both hypothyroidism and hyperthyroidism.

10. Swelling in the neck: Enlargement of the thyroid gland, known as a goiter, may cause visible swelling in the front of the neck.

It's important to note that these symptoms can be caused by various other factors as well, and experiencing one or more of these signs does not necessarily mean you have a thyroid disorder. Proper diagnosis requires medical evaluation and testing by a healthcare professional. If you suspect you have a thyroid disorder, it is advisable to seek medical advice for accurate diagnosis and appropriate treatment.

## Common Thyroid Disorder

There are several common thyroid disorders that affect the functioning of the thyroid gland. Here are a few of them:

1. Hypothyroidism: This is a condition in which the thyroid gland does not produce enough thyroid hormones. It can result in a slower metabolism and lead to symptoms such as fatigue, weight gain, cold intolerance, depression, dry skin, and constipation.

2. Hyperthyroidism: This condition occurs when the thyroid gland produces an excess of thyroid hormones. It can cause an overactive metabolism, resulting in symptoms such as weight loss, increased appetite, rapid heartbeat, anxiety, irritability, tremors, heat intolerance, and difficulty sleeping.

3. Thyroid nodules: Thyroid nodules are lumps or abnormal growths that form within the thyroid gland. They can be solid or fluid-filled and may be benign (noncancerous) or cancerous. Thyroid nodules may not cause any symptoms, but larger

nodules can lead to difficulty swallowing, hoarseness, or visible swelling in the neck.

4. Thyroiditis: Thyroiditis refers to inflammation of the thyroid gland. It can occur due to various causes, including autoimmune conditions, viral infections, or medications. Thyroiditis can cause temporary hyperthyroidism, followed by hypothyroidism or a return to normal thyroid function.

5. Hashimoto's thyroiditis: It is an autoimmune condition where the immune system attacks the thyroid gland, leading to chronic inflammation and gradual destruction of thyroid tissue. Hashimoto's thyroiditis is the most common cause of hypothyroidism and can result in fatigue, depression, weight gain, muscle weakness, and sensitivity to cold.

These are just a few examples of common thyroid disorders. It's important to consult a healthcare professional for proper diagnosis and management if you suspect you have a thyroid condition. They can provide a comprehensive evaluation, perform necessary tests, and recommend appropriate treatment options.

## Treatment Of Thyroid Disorder

The treatment of thyroid disorders depends on the specific condition and its underlying cause. Here are some common treatment approaches for different thyroid disorders:

1. Hypothyroidism:
   - Synthetic thyroid hormone replacement: The primary treatment for hypothyroidism is taking synthetic thyroid hormone medication, such as levothyroxine. This medication helps to restore normal thyroid hormone levels in the body.

2. Hyperthyroidism:
   - Antithyroid medications: Medications like methimazole or propylthiouracil may be prescribed to reduce the production of thyroid hormones.

- Radioactive iodine therapy: This treatment involves taking a radioactive iodine pill, which selectively destroys the overactive thyroid cells.
- Thyroidectomy: Surgical removal of the thyroid gland may be recommended in certain cases, especially if medications and radioactive iodine therapy are not effective or contraindicated.

3. Thyroid nodules:
- Observation: Small, benign nodules may not require treatment but will be monitored over time.
- Fine-needle aspiration biopsy: If a nodule is suspicious, a small sample of cells may be taken for testing to determine if further treatment or monitoring is needed.
- Surgery: Surgical removal of the nodule or the entire thyroid gland may be recommended in certain cases, such as when the nodule is cancerous or causing symptoms.

4. Thyroiditis:
- Treatment of underlying cause: Depending on the specific type of thyroiditis, treatment may involve managing symptoms, anti-inflammatory

medications, or addressing underlying infections or autoimmune conditions.

It's important to note that treatment plans are personalized for each individual, and the approach may vary based on factors such as the severity of the condition, age, overall health, and patient preferences. Regular monitoring of thyroid hormone levels and follow-up with a healthcare professional is typically required to ensure optimal management of thyroid disorders.

It's always recommended to consult with a healthcare professional for a proper diagnosis and individualized treatment plan based on your specific thyroid condition.

# CHAPTER TWO: Thyroid Bolster Recipe

## How does it work

The phrase "thyroid bolster recipe" suggests a recipe that is specifically designed to support or enhance the health and function of the thyroid gland. While there is no specific food or recipe that can directly cure or treat thyroid disorders, a thyroid bolster recipe would typically focus on including ingredients that are beneficial for thyroid health.

Here's how a thyroid bolster recipe might work:

1. Nutrient-rich ingredients: The recipe would likely include foods that are rich in essential nutrients for thyroid function. This may include foods high in iodine (such as seaweed), selenium (such as Brazil nuts), zinc, and vitamins A, D, and E. These nutrients are important for thyroid hormone production and metabolism.

2. Anti-inflammatory ingredients: Many thyroid disorders involve inflammation, so a thyroid bolster recipe may incorporate ingredients known for their anti-inflammatory properties. This could include foods like fatty fish (rich in omega-3 fatty acids), turmeric, ginger, leafy greens, and berries.

3. Balanced macronutrients: The recipe would likely provide a balanced combination of carbohydrates, proteins, and healthy fats. This balance helps maintain stable blood sugar levels and provides sustained energy, which can be beneficial for overall thyroid health.

4. Fiber-rich ingredients: Including fiber-rich ingredients, such as whole grains, legumes, and vegetables, can support digestion and help regulate blood sugar levels, which is important for individuals with thyroid disorders.

5. Avoiding potential triggers: Depending on the specific thyroid condition, certain ingredients or foods may need to be avoided. For example, individuals with hypothyroidism may need to limit

goitrogenic foods (such as cruciferous vegetables) that can interfere with thyroid function.

It's important to note that a thyroid bolster recipe should be part of an overall balanced and varied diet, and it should not replace medical treatment or advice. It's always recommended to consult with a healthcare professional or a registered dietitian for personalized guidance and to ensure that any dietary changes align with your specific health needs and condition.

## Thyroid Friendly Food

When it comes to supporting thyroid health, including certain foods in your diet can be beneficial. While no single food can cure thyroid disorders, incorporating these thyroid-friendly foods can provide essential nutrients and support overall well-being. Here are some examples:

1. Iodine-rich foods: Iodine is a crucial nutrient for thyroid hormone production. Good sources include

seaweed (such as kelp and nori), iodized salt, seafood (like fish and shrimp), and dairy products.

2. Selenium-rich foods: Selenium is important for thyroid hormone metabolism and function. Foods rich in selenium include Brazil nuts, sardines, tuna, eggs, legumes, and whole grains.

3. Omega-3 fatty acids: Found in fatty fish (such as salmon, mackerel, and sardines), flaxseeds, chia seeds, and walnuts, omega-3 fatty acids have anti-inflammatory properties and may help reduce inflammation associated with thyroid disorders.

4. Antioxidant-rich fruits and vegetables: Fruits and vegetables are abundant in antioxidants that help combat oxidative stress. Include a variety of colorful options like berries, leafy greens, bell peppers, carrots, and tomatoes.

5. Zinc-containing foods: Zinc is important for thyroid hormone production and metabolism. Foods rich in zinc include oysters, beef, poultry, pumpkin seeds, nuts, and legumes.

6. Vitamin D sources: Adequate vitamin D levels are linked to better thyroid function. Get natural sunlight exposure and include vitamin D-rich foods such as fatty fish, fortified dairy products, and egg yolks in your diet.

7. Gluten-free grains: Some individuals with autoimmune thyroid conditions find relief by adopting a gluten-free diet. Consider incorporating gluten-free grains like quinoa, rice, buckwheat, and amaranth.

8. Fermented foods: Gut health is closely linked to thyroid health. Fermented foods like yogurt, kefir, sauerkraut, and kimchi can support a healthy gut microbiome.

Remember, individual dietary needs may vary, and it's important to consult with a healthcare professional or a registered dietitian for personalized guidance based on your specific thyroid condition. They can provide appropriate recommendations tailored to your needs and help you maintain a well-balanced diet.

## Food to Avoid For Healthy Thyroid

While certain foods can be beneficial for thyroid health, it's also important to be aware of foods that may interfere with thyroid function or exacerbate certain thyroid conditions. Here are some foods that some individuals with thyroid disorders may consider avoiding or limiting:

1. Goitrogenic foods: Some foods contain compounds called goitrogens that can interfere with thyroid function by blocking iodine uptake or inhibiting the production of thyroid hormones. Examples of goitrogenic foods include cruciferous vegetables (such as broccoli, cauliflower, cabbage, kale, and Brussels sprouts), soy products, millet, and certain fruits like peaches and strawberries. However, cooking these foods can help reduce their goitrogenic effects.

2. Gluten: Some individuals with autoimmune thyroid conditions, such as Hashimoto's thyroiditis, may benefit from avoiding gluten-containing grains like wheat, barley, and rye. Gluten may trigger an immune response and contribute to inflammation in susceptible individuals.

3. Excessive iodine: While iodine is essential for thyroid health, excessive intake of iodine can be detrimental, especially for individuals with certain thyroid conditions. Excess iodine may aggravate hyperthyroidism and autoimmune thyroid disorders. It's important to consult with a healthcare professional to determine the appropriate iodine intake for your specific condition.

4. High-sugar and processed foods: A diet high in refined sugars, processed foods, and unhealthy fats can contribute to inflammation and disrupt overall hormonal balance, including thyroid function. Limiting these foods and opting for whole, nutrient-dense options is generally beneficial for overall health, including thyroid health.

5. Excessive caffeine: While moderate caffeine intake is generally well-tolerated, excessive consumption of caffeine from sources like coffee, tea, energy drinks, and sodas can interfere with thyroid hormone absorption and exacerbate symptoms of hyperthyroidism.

6. Alcohol: Alcohol can interfere with thyroid hormone production and metabolism. It may also disrupt the conversion of T4 to T3, affecting thyroid function. Moderate alcohol consumption is generally recommended if you have a healthy thyroid, but it's advisable to consult with your healthcare professional for specific guidance if you have a thyroid disorder.

It's important to note that individual sensitivities and responses to these foods can vary. Not everyone with a thyroid disorder will need to avoid these foods entirely. It's recommended to work with a healthcare professional or a registered dietitian who specializes in thyroid health to determine the most appropriate dietary approach for your specific condition. They can provide personalized recommendations based on your individual needs and help you make informed choices for a healthier thyroid.

## One Week Thyroid Bolster Recipe Plan

Here's a one-week meal plan for supporting a healthy thyroid:

Day 1:
- Breakfast: Veggie omelet with spinach, mushrooms, and tomatoes.
- Lunch: Quinoa salad with mixed vegetables, chickpeas, and a lemon-tahini dressing.
- Dinner: Baked salmon with steamed broccoli and a side of quinoa.
- Snack: Greek yogurt with berries and a sprinkle of chia seeds.

Day 2:
- Breakfast: Overnight oats with almond milk, sliced banana, and a dollop of almond butter.

- Lunch: Mixed greens salad with grilled chicken, avocado, cherry tomatoes, and balsamic vinaigrette.
- Dinner: Roasted chicken breast with roasted sweet potatoes and steamed asparagus.
- Snack: Carrot sticks with hummus.

Day 3:
- Breakfast: Smoothie made with almond milk, spinach, banana, and a scoop of protein powder.
- Lunch: Lentil soup with a side of mixed greens salad.
- Dinner: Stir-fried tofu with mixed vegetables and brown rice.
- Snack: Handful of almonds and an apple.

Day 4:
- Breakfast: Greek yogurt with sliced peaches and a sprinkle of granola.
- Lunch: Quinoa and black bean salad with roasted vegetables and a lime-cilantro dressing.
- Dinner: Grilled chicken or tempeh with roasted Brussels sprouts and quinoa.
- Snack: Celery sticks with almond butter.

Day 5:
- Breakfast: Scrambled eggs with sautéed spinach and cherry tomatoes.
- Lunch: Chickpea and vegetable curry with brown rice.
- Dinner: Baked cod with roasted cauliflower and a side of quinoa.
- Snack: Mixed berries with a handful of walnuts.

Please note that this meal plan is a general guideline and may need to be adjusted based on individual dietary needs and preferences. It's always a good idea to consult with a healthcare professional or a registered dietitian for personalized advice.

# CHAPTER THREE: Amazing Thyroid Bolster Recipe

## Meat Recipe

### Barbecued Beef

Barbecue beef is a popular dish that involves grilling or smoking beef cuts, typically marinated in a flavorful sauce or dry rub. The beef is slow-cooked over low heat, resulting in tender, juicy meat with a smoky and caramelized exterior. Barbecue beef is known for its rich and savory flavor profile, often enhanced by various spices, herbs, and tangy barbecue sauces. It is a beloved dish enjoyed at cookouts, picnics, and gatherings, offering a delicious and satisfying dining experience for meat lovers.

### Beef and Mushroom Stew

Beef and mushroom stew is a hearty and comforting dish that combines tender beef chunks with earthy mushrooms in a flavorful broth. The beef is typically seared to develop a rich caramelized exterior, then simmered with mushrooms, onions, garlic, and aromatic herbs and spices. The stew slowly cooks, allowing the flavors to meld together and the beef to become tender and juicy. The addition of mushrooms adds depth and a unique umami flavor to the stew. This dish is often served with crusty bread or over mashed potatoes, creating a satisfying meal for chilly days or whenever you crave a comforting, savory dish.

## Peasant Soup

Peasant soup is a simple and rustic dish that has its roots in traditional, hearty cooking. It typically consists of a variety of vegetables, legumes, and sometimes meat or poultry, simmered together in a flavorful broth. The ingredients used in peasant soup can vary based on regional and seasonal availability. This soup is known for its humble ingredients and comforting flavors, making it a nourishing and satisfying meal. Peasant soup is often enjoyed during colder months or whenever a warm and wholesome dish is desired.

## Eggplant Stew

Eggplant stew is a flavorful and hearty dish that showcases the versatility of eggplants. This stew typically combines tender chunks of eggplant with onions, garlic, tomatoes, and a variety of herbs and spices. The eggplant absorbs the flavors of the ingredients, resulting in a rich and savory stew. Sometimes, additional vegetables, legumes, or protein sources like chickpeas or tofu are added to enhance the dish. Eggplant stew can be enjoyed as a standalone meal or served over rice or with crusty bread. It offers a delicious and satisfying option for vegetarians or anyone looking to explore the unique flavors of eggplants in a comforting stew.

## Irish Stew

Irish stew is a traditional and iconic dish hailing from Ireland. It is a simple yet hearty one-pot meal that typically consists of lamb or mutton, potatoes, onions, carrots, and herbs. The stew is slow-cooked, allowing the flavors to meld together and the meat to become tender and flavorful. The combination of meat, root vegetables, and aromatic herbs creates a comforting and nourishing dish, perfect for cold weather or a hearty meal. Irish stew is a staple in Irish cuisine and continues to be enjoyed as a classic and satisfying dish worldwide.

## Grilled Lamb

Grilled lamb is a succulent and flavorful dish that showcases the unique taste of lamb meat. It involves cooking lamb cuts, such as chops or racks, over an open flame or on a grill. The lamb is typically marinated with herbs, spices, and sometimes a tangy sauce to enhance its natural flavors. Grilling lamb imparts a smoky char and caramelization on the outside while keeping the meat juicy and tender on the inside. The result is a delicious and satisfying dish that is often enjoyed as a centerpiece at special occasions or as part of a hearty meal. Grilled lamb is a popular choice for meat lovers seeking a rich and savory dining experience.

## Stuffed Banana peppers

Stuffed banana peppers are a delicious and savory dish that features mild or hot banana peppers filled with a flavorful stuffing. The peppers are typically slit lengthwise and seeded before being stuffed with a mixture of ingredients such as cheese, breadcrumbs, herbs, and sometimes meat or vegetables. The stuffed peppers are then baked or grilled until the peppers are tender and the filling is golden and melted. The combination of the slightly sweet and tangy banana peppers with the savory stuffing creates a delightful contrast of flavors. Stuffed banana peppers can be enjoyed as an appetizer, side dish, or even as a main course, offering a tasty and satisfying option for those who enjoy a bit of spice and a burst of flavor.

# Chicken and Poultry Recipes

## Lemon Herb Roast Chicken

Lemon Herb Roast Chicken is a classic and flavorful dish that involves rubbing a whole chicken with a mixture of lemon zest, minced garlic, fresh herbs, salt, and pepper. The chicken is then roasted in the oven until the skin becomes golden and crispy, while the meat remains juicy and tender. The combination of zesty lemon, aromatic herbs, and savory flavors creates a delicious and aromatic roast chicken. This dish is perfect for a Sunday dinner or any special occasion, and it pairs well with roasted vegetables or a fresh salad. Lemon Herb Roast Chicken offers a delightful balance of tanginess and herb-infused richness that is sure to please chicken lovers.

## Honey Mustard Glazed Chicken Thighs

Honey Mustard Glazed Chicken Thighs are a delicious and savory dish that features tender chicken thighs coated in a sweet and tangy glaze. The glaze is made by combining honey, Dijon mustard, minced garlic, soy sauce, and a squeeze of lemon juice. The chicken thighs are then coated in the glaze and baked until they are cooked through and the glaze becomes caramelized and slightly sticky. The combination of the sweet honey, tangy mustard, and savory flavors creates a delightful balance of tastes. Honey Mustard Glazed Chicken Thighs are an easy and flavorful option for a weeknight dinner, and they pair well with steamed rice and vegetables.

## Turkey Meatball

Turkey meatballs are a delicious and healthier alternative to traditional meatballs, made using ground turkey instead of beef. The ground turkey is combined with breadcrumbs, grated Parmesan cheese, minced garlic, chopped parsley, salt, and pepper to form flavorful meatballs. These meatballs are then baked in the oven until they are cooked through and slightly browned. Turkey meatballs offer a lighter and leaner option while still providing a savory and satisfying taste. They can be served with marinara sauce and pasta, on a sub roll for sandwiches, or even as an appetizer. Turkey meatballs are a versatile and flavorful choice for those looking for a leaner meatball option.

## Grilled Lemon Pepper Chicken Skewers

Grilled lemon pepper chicken skewers are a flavorful and easy-to-make dish that features marinated chicken chunks threaded onto skewers and grilled to perfection. The chicken is marinated in a mixture of lemon juice, olive oil, minced garlic, and cracked black pepper, which infuses it with tangy and aromatic flavors. Grilling the skewers gives the chicken a charred and smoky taste while keeping it tender and juicy. Grilled lemon pepper chicken skewers are versatile and can be served as a main course or as part of a salad or wrap. They offer a delightful combination of zesty lemon, bold pepper, and succulent grilled chicken, making them a delicious and satisfying option for any occasion.

## Baked Parmesan Chicken

Baked Parmesan chicken is a flavorful and easy-to-make dish that involves coating boneless, skinless chicken breasts in a mixture of grated Parmesan cheese, breadcrumbs, garlic powder, and Italian seasoning. The chicken is then baked in the oven until it becomes golden and crispy on the outside and cooked through on the inside. The combination of the Parmesan cheese and seasonings adds a savory and cheesy taste to the chicken, making it a crowd-pleasing dish. Baked Parmesan chicken can be served with a side of marinara sauce and pasta or alongside steamed vegetables for a complete and delicious meal.

## Chicken Salad

Chicken salad is a refreshing and versatile dish that combines cooked chicken with a variety of ingredients. The cooked chicken is typically shredded or diced and mixed with mayonnaise, along with additions such as celery, onions, grapes, apples, nuts, or herbs. The salad can be customized with different flavors and textures to suit personal preferences. Chicken salad is often served chilled and can be enjoyed on its own, as a sandwich filling, or as a topping for greens. It offers a light and protein-packed option for a quick and satisfying meal, perfect for picnics, lunches, or gatherings.

## Chili Pronto

Chili Pronto is a quick and easy version of chili that can be prepared in a short amount of time. It typically involves browning ground beef or turkey with onions and garlic, then adding canned beans, diced tomatoes, and a blend of chili spices. The mixture is simmered until the flavors meld together and the chili thickens. Chili Pronto offers a hearty and flavorful meal that can be customized with additional ingredients such as bell peppers, corn, or jalapeños for added texture and heat. It is a popular dish enjoyed during colder months or whenever a comforting and satisfying bowl of chili is desired.

## Chicken salad with orange juice

Chicken salad with orange juice is a refreshing and citrusy twist on the classic chicken salad. It typically involves combining cooked and shredded chicken with a variety of ingredients such as mayonnaise, diced celery, chopped onions, and seasonings. The addition of orange juice adds a tangy and bright flavor to the salad, giving it a refreshing taste. The orange juice can be incorporated into the dressing or used to marinate the chicken beforehand to infuse it with citrus notes. Chicken salad with orange juice is a delightful option for those who enjoy a zesty and vibrant twist to their salads. It can be served on a bed of lettuce, in a sandwich, or as a light and flavorful side dish.

## Corn and salsa chicken salad

Salsa chicken salad with corn is a delicious and vibrant dish that combines the flavors of salsa, chicken, and sweet corn. It typically involves cooking chicken breasts and shredding them, then mixing them with salsa, corn kernels, diced tomatoes, chopped bell peppers, and other desired ingredients. The salsa adds a tangy and spicy kick to the salad, while the corn provides a touch of sweetness and crunch. This chicken salad variation offers a unique twist with its bold and zesty flavors. It can be served on a bed of lettuce, in tortillas as a wrap, or as a flavorful topping for nachos or tacos. Salsa chicken salad with corn is a versatile and satisfying option for those who enjoy a combination of fresh ingredients and bold flavors.

## Easy chicken Lasagna

Easy chicken lasagna is a simplified version of the classic Italian dish that substitutes traditional ground meat with cooked chicken. It typically involves layering lasagna noodles, cooked chicken, marinara sauce, ricotta or cottage cheese, and mozzarella cheese in a baking dish. The layers are repeated until the dish is filled, and it's then baked until the cheese is melted and bubbly. This variation offers a lighter and flavorful twist to traditional lasagna. Easy chicken lasagna is a convenient and delicious option for a comforting family meal or for those who prefer poultry over beef or pork. It can be served with a side salad or garlic bread for a complete and satisfying dinner.

# Fish and Seafood Recipes

## Grilled Salmon with Lemon and Dill

Grilled salmon with lemon and dill is a simple and flavorful dish that showcases the natural taste of salmon. The salmon fillets are seasoned with salt, pepper, fresh lemon juice, and chopped dill. They are then grilled over medium-high heat until cooked through and slightly charred on the edges. The combination of zesty lemon, aromatic dill, and perfectly grilled salmon creates a delightful balance of flavors. Grilled salmon with lemon and dill is a popular choice for seafood lovers seeking a light and refreshing dish. It can be served as a main course alongside steamed vegetables or a fresh salad, offering a healthy and delicious meal option.

## Fish Tacos

Fish tacos are a popular and delicious dish that combines crispy or grilled fish with flavorful toppings, wrapped in a soft tortilla. The fish, often a white flaky variety like cod or tilapia, is seasoned and cooked until tender. The tortillas are warmed and filled with the cooked fish, along with toppings like shredded lettuce, diced tomatoes, avocado slices, and a squeeze of lime juice. Additional condiments such as salsa, sour cream, or a tangy sauce can be added for extra flavor. Fish tacos offer a delightful combination of textures and flavors, with the fresh ingredients complementing the succulent fish. They are a versatile and enjoyable meal option that can be easily customized to personal taste preferences.

## Shrimp Scampi

Shrimp scampi is a classic and mouth watering dish that features plump shrimp cooked in a flavorful garlic and butter sauce. The peeled and deveined shrimp are sautéed in a combination of butter, minced garlic, and a splash of white wine, which enhances the savory flavors. Fresh lemon juice, red pepper flakes, and chopped parsley are added to the pan to create a delightful balance of tanginess and heat. Shrimp scampi is typically served over cooked pasta, allowing the pasta to soak up the delicious sauce. It's a quick and easy recipe that delivers a burst of flavors, making it a favorite choice for seafood lovers.

## Grilled Lemon Herb Sea Bass

Grilled lemon herb sea bass is a light and flavorful dish that features tender sea bass fillets marinated in a blend of fresh lemon juice and a mixture of chopped herbs such as thyme, rosemary, and parsley. The sea bass is then grilled over medium heat until it's cooked through, resulting in a delicate and flaky texture. The combination of zesty lemon, aromatic herbs, and perfectly grilled sea bass creates a harmonious medley of flavors. Grilled lemon herb sea bass is a popular choice for seafood enthusiasts seeking a healthy and delicious meal. It pairs well with a drizzle of olive oil and additional fresh herbs for garnish, making it a delightful and visually appealing dish.

## Garlic Butter Shrimp

Garlic butter shrimp is a quick and flavorful dish that highlights the natural sweetness of shrimp. The peeled and deveined shrimp are cooked in a mixture of melted butter, minced garlic, and chopped parsley. The garlic infuses the shrimp with a rich and savory flavor, while the butter adds a luscious and indulgent touch. The shrimp are cooked until they turn pink and are tender. Garlic butter shrimp can be served as an appetizer, tossed with pasta, or enjoyed as a main course. It's a versatile dish that is loved for its simplicity and deliciousness.

## Mussels Mariniere

Mussels Mariniere is a classic French dish that features fresh mussels cooked in a flavorful broth. The mussels are steamed in a fragrant combination of white wine, garlic, shallots, and parsley, which infuses them with a delicate and savory taste. The dish is typically finished with a knob of butter to add richness and silkiness to the broth. Mussels Mariniere is served with crusty bread to soak up the flavorful broth and enjoy the tender mussels. It is a beloved seafood dish known for its simplicity and the wonderful flavors that come from the combination of ingredients.

## Maple Salmon

Maple salmon is a delectable dish that showcases the natural sweetness of salmon complemented by a rich and sticky maple glaze. The salmon fillets are coated in a mixture of maple syrup, soy sauce, minced garlic, and a touch of Dijon mustard. The fish is then baked or grilled until it's cooked through and the glaze becomes caramelized, resulting in a perfect balance of sweet and savory flavors. Maple salmon is a favorite choice for seafood enthusiasts seeking a delightful and easy-to-make meal. It pairs well with a side of steamed vegetables or rice, offering a satisfying and delicious dining experience.

## Baked Coconut Shrimp

Baked coconut shrimp is a delightful dish that features large shrimp coated in a crispy and flavorful coconut crust. The shrimp are first dipped in a mixture of flour, egg, and seasonings, then coated in shredded coconut. They are then baked in the oven until the coconut coating turns golden brown and crispy. Baking the shrimp instead of frying them reduces the oil content while still achieving a satisfying texture. Baked coconut shrimp is often served as an appetizer or as part of a main course. The combination of the succulent shrimp and the sweet and nutty flavor of the coconut creates a tropical and irresistible treat.

## Rice and Tuna Salad

Rice and tuna salad is a delicious and satisfying dish that combines cooked rice, flaked tuna, and an assortment of fresh vegetables and herbs. The salad is typically dressed with a tangy vinaigrette or a creamy dressing, which adds flavor and helps bring all the ingredients together. Additional ingredients such as diced cucumbers, cherry tomatoes, chopped onions, and herbs like parsley or dill are often included to enhance the salad's texture and taste. Rice and tuna salad can be enjoyed as a standalone meal or served as a filling for sandwiches or wraps. It offers a nutritious and versatile option that is perfect for picnics, lunches, or quick and easy dinners.

# Vegan and Vegetarian Recipes

## Quinoa Porridge

Quinoa porridge is a nutritious and comforting breakfast dish made with quinoa grains. It is a healthy alternative to traditional oatmeal and provides a good source of protein, fiber, and essential nutrients. To make quinoa porridge, rinse the quinoa thoroughly, then cook it with water or plant-based milk until it becomes soft and the liquid is absorbed. Add sweeteners like maple syrup or honey, as well as toppings such as fresh fruits, nuts, and seeds for added flavor and texture. Quinoa porridge offers a warm and satisfying start to the day and is a popular choice among those seeking a gluten-free and nutrient-rich breakfast option.

## Seaweed Salad

Seaweed salad is a refreshing and nutritious dish made from various types of edible seaweed. The seaweed is typically soaked and then dressed with a mixture of soy sauce, rice vinegar, sesame oil, and other seasonings like ginger and garlic. It is often garnished with sesame seeds or sliced vegetables for added texture and flavor. Seaweed salad is known for its unique combination of salty, umami, and slightly briny taste. It is enjoyed as a side dish or appetizer in many Asian cuisines and is appreciated for its health benefits, including being a good source of minerals and antioxidants. Seaweed salad offers a delightful and light addition to a balanced meal.

## Spinach with Mushroom

Spinach with mushrooms is a simple and nutritious dish that combines the earthy flavors of mushrooms with the vibrant green goodness of spinach. The dish typically involves sautéing sliced mushrooms and minced garlic in a bit of olive oil until the mushrooms are tender and golden brown. Fresh spinach leaves are then added to the pan and cooked until they wilt. The combination of the tender mushrooms and the delicate spinach creates a delightful contrast in textures. Spinach with mushrooms can be enjoyed as a side dish or served over rice, pasta, or as a filling for sandwiches or wraps. It's a versatile and healthy option that provides a satisfying dose of vitamins, minerals, and fiber.

## Avocado and Mango

Avocado and mango is a delightful combination that brings together the creamy richness of avocado with the sweet and juicy flavors of mango. When combined, they create a harmonious blend of textures and tastes. Avocado provides a smooth and buttery texture, while mango adds a refreshing and tropical sweetness. The combination works well in salads, salsas, smoothies, and even on toast. Avocado and mango are not only delicious but also offer a range of health benefits. Avocado is a good source of healthy fats, fiber, and vitamins, while mango is rich in antioxidants, vitamins, and minerals. Together, they make a delicious and nutritious pairing that adds a burst of flavor to various dishes.

## Black Beans

Black beans are a versatile and nutritious legume that are commonly used in various cuisines around the world. They have a dense and meaty texture, along with a rich and earthy flavor. Black beans are an excellent source of plant-based protein, fiber, vitamins, and minerals. They can be cooked and used in a variety of dishes, including soups, stews, salads, burritos, and dips. Black beans are a staple in many vegetarian and vegan diets due to their nutritional profile and ability to add depth and substance to meals. They are also known for their potential health benefits, such as supporting heart health and aiding digestion. Incorporating black beans into your diet is a delicious and nutritious way to enjoy a plant-based protein source.

## Vegan Chickpea Salad Sandwich

A vegan chickpea salad sandwich is a flavorful and satisfying alternative to traditional chicken or tuna salad sandwiches. It involves mashing cooked chickpeas and mixing them with vegan mayo or tahini, along with ingredients like diced celery, red onion, pickles, and seasonings such as lemon juice, mustard, and herbs. The mixture is then spread onto bread or wraps and can be further enhanced with lettuce, tomato slices, or avocado. This plant-based sandwich option offers a good source of protein and fiber from the chickpeas, while the combination of flavors and textures creates a delicious and filling meal. Vegan chickpea salad sandwiches are a popular choice for those seeking a cruelty-free and nutritious sandwich option.

## Vegan Lentil Curry

Vegan lentil curry is a flavorful and hearty dish made with lentils and an array of spices and vegetables. It involves simmering cooked lentils in a fragrant curry sauce that typically includes ingredients such as onions, garlic, ginger, and a blend of spices like cumin, turmeric, coriander, and chili powder. Additional vegetables like tomatoes, spinach, or bell peppers can be added to enhance the dish's nutritional value. Vegan lentil curry is known for its rich and aromatic flavors, as well as its high protein and fiber content from the lentils. It is often served with rice or naan bread, making it a satisfying and nourishing meal option for those following a plant-based diet.

## Vegetarian Chill

Vegetarian chili is a delicious and satisfying meat-free version of the classic chili dish. It is made with a combination of beans, vegetables, and flavorful spices. Common ingredients include kidney beans, black beans, tomatoes, onions, bell peppers, and a variety of chili seasonings like chili powder, cumin, paprika, and oregano. Vegetarian chili is known for its hearty and robust flavors, and it can be customized with additional vegetables, such as corn or zucchini, for added texture and taste. It is a nutritious option packed with protein and fiber from the beans and plenty of vitamins and antioxidants from the vegetables. Vegetarian chili is a favorite among both vegetarians and meat-eaters, as it offers a satisfying and flavorful meal that can be enjoyed on its own or served with rice, tortilla chips, or a side of crusty bread.

## Vegetables Tangine

Vegetable tagine is a flavorful and aromatic Moroccan dish that combines a variety of vegetables cooked in a rich and fragrant sauce. Traditional tagine recipes often feature vegetables such as carrots, potatoes, eggplant, bell peppers, and tomatoes. The dish is seasoned with a blend of spices like cumin, coriander, turmeric, cinnamon, and paprika, which infuse the vegetables with a warm and savory taste. The vegetables are typically slow-cooked in a tagine pot or a similar covered cooking vessel, allowing the flavors to meld together and the vegetables to become tender. Vegetable tagine is a versatile and nutritious dish that can be enjoyed on its own or served with couscous, rice, or bread. It offers a vibrant and satisfying option for both vegetarians and vegans, highlighting the natural flavors of the vegetables and the aromatic spices of Moroccan cuisine.

# Stew and Soup

## Paleo Chicken Soup

Paleo chicken soup is a nourishing and comforting soup made with chicken and a variety of vegetables. It follows the principles of the Paleo diet, which focuses on consuming whole, unprocessed foods. In this recipe, chicken is simmered in a broth with vegetables such as carrots, celery, onions, and herbs like thyme or rosemary. The result is a flavorful and nutrient-dense soup that is free from grains, dairy, and legumes. It provides a good source of protein, healthy fats, and vitamins. Paleo chicken soup is a warming and satisfying option for those following a Paleo lifestyle or anyone seeking a wholesome and nourishing meal.

## Tomato Curry Lentil Stew

Tomato curry lentil stew is a hearty and flavorful dish that combines the richness of lentils with the tanginess of tomatoes and aromatic curry spices. The stew is typically made by simmering lentils in a tomato-based broth along with onions, garlic, ginger, and a blend of curry spices like cumin, coriander, turmeric, and garam masala. The lentils absorb the flavors of the spices and the tangy sweetness of the tomatoes, resulting in a delicious and satisfying stew. This dish is not only packed with plant-based protein and fiber from the lentils but also offers a range of vitamins and minerals from the vegetables and spices. Tomato curry lentil stew is a nourishing and comforting choice for those looking to enjoy a vegetarian or vegan meal with robust flavors and wholesome ingredients.

## White Bean Chicken Chili

White bean chicken chili is a comforting and flavorful soup that combines tender chicken, white beans, and aromatic spices. The dish typically involves sautéing onions, garlic, and diced chicken until cooked through. White beans, such as cannellini or Great Northern beans, are then added to the pot along with chicken broth, green chilies, and seasonings like cumin, oregano, and chili powder. The chili is simmered until the flavors meld together, creating a hearty and satisfying soup. White bean chicken chili offers a good source of protein from the chicken and beans, while the combination of spices adds a delightful kick. It's a delicious and nourishing option for those seeking a comforting and protein-rich meal.

## Chickpea and Spanish Spinach Stew

Chickpea and spinach stew is a flavorful and nutritious dish that combines the earthy taste of chickpeas with the vibrant flavors of Spanish cuisine. The stew is made by sautéing onions, garlic, and spices like paprika and cumin in a pot. Chickpeas, diced tomatoes, and vegetable broth are then added, and the stew is simmered until the flavors meld together. Fresh spinach leaves are stirred in at the end, wilting slightly and adding a pop of vibrant green color. This stew is rich in plant-based protein and fiber from the chickpeas, while the combination of spices and vegetables provides a depth of flavor. Chickpea and spinach stew is a hearty and satisfying option that can be enjoyed on its own or served over rice or with crusty bread. It offers a delightful taste of Spain with a healthy twist.

## Vegetables Lentil Soup

Vegetable lentil soup is a nourishing and flavorful dish that combines the goodness of lentils with a variety of vegetables. This soup typically includes ingredients like onions, carrots, celery, bell peppers, and tomatoes, along with lentils and a vegetable broth or stock. It is seasoned with herbs and spices like thyme, rosemary, cumin, and paprika, which infuse the soup with a delightful aroma and taste. The lentils provide a good source of plant-based protein and fiber, while the vegetables contribute vitamins, minerals, and antioxidants. Vegetable lentil soup is a comforting and satisfying option that can be enjoyed as a standalone meal or served with crusty bread. It's a nutritious choice for those seeking a hearty and wholesome soup packed with vegetables and lentils.

## Classic Tomato soup

Classic tomato soup is a comforting and timeless dish made with ripe tomatoes, onions, garlic, and a few simple seasonings. The soup is typically prepared by sautéing onions and garlic until fragrant, then adding tomatoes (fresh or canned) and simmering until they break down. The mixture is then blended until smooth, resulting in a velvety texture. The soup is often enriched with a splash of cream or milk for added richness. Classic tomato soup is known for its tangy and savory flavor, and it pairs perfectly with grilled cheese sandwiches or crusty bread. It is a versatile and beloved favorite that can be enjoyed all year round.

## Butternut squash Soup

Butternut squash soup is a creamy and comforting soup made from roasted or cooked butternut squash. The soup typically involves sautéing onions and garlic, adding diced butternut squash, vegetable broth, and spices like nutmeg, cinnamon, and a touch of maple syrup or honey for sweetness. The mixture is simmered until the squash is tender and then blended until smooth, creating a velvety texture. Butternut squash soup is known for its rich and earthy flavor, as well as its vibrant orange color. It is a nutritious option, packed with vitamins, minerals, and fiber from the squash. This soup is often served as an appetizer or as a main dish, and it pairs well with a garnish of fresh herbs or a sprinkle of toasted pumpkin seeds. It is a delicious and satisfying choice for fall and winter seasons.

## Pasta Fagioli

Pasta fagioli is a hearty Italian soup that combines pasta and beans in a flavorful tomato-based broth. The soup typically includes ingredients like onions, garlic, carrots, celery, diced tomatoes, cannellini beans, and small pasta such as ditalini or macaroni. It is seasoned with herbs like oregano, basil, and thyme, along with a touch of red pepper flakes for a hint of spice. The pasta absorbs the flavors of the broth, while the beans add a creamy texture and a good source of plant-based protein and fiber. Pasta fagioli is a comforting and satisfying soup that can be enjoyed on its own or served with a sprinkle of grated Parmesan cheese and crusty bread. It's a classic Italian dish that is both flavorful and nourishing.

## Vegan Buddha Bowl

A Vegan Buddha Bowl is a nourishing and balanced meal consisting of various plant-based ingredients arranged in a bowl. It typically includes a combination of cooked grains like quinoa or brown rice, roasted or sautéed vegetables, legumes such as chickpeas or black beans, and fresh greens. The bowl is often topped with a flavorful dressing or sauce for added taste. Vegan Buddha Bowls are not only visually appealing but also provide a wide array of nutrients, including protein, fiber, vitamins, and minerals. They offer versatility in ingredient choices, allowing individuals to customize their bowls to their taste preferences and dietary needs. Enjoy the vibrant colors, textures, and flavors of a Vegan Buddha Bowl as a wholesome and satisfying meal.

## Lentil and Vegetable Stir-Fry

Lentil and Vegetable Stir-Fry is a nutritious and flavorful dish that combines protein-rich lentils with a colorful assortment of vegetables. The stir-fry typically includes ingredients such as cooked lentils, bell peppers, carrots, broccoli, onions, and garlic, along with a savory sauce made from soy sauce, ginger, and other seasonings. The dish is quickly cooked in a hot pan or wok, allowing the vegetables to retain their crispness and the lentils to absorb the flavors of the sauce. Lentil and Vegetable Stir-Fry is a versatile and satisfying meal, providing a good balance of protein, fiber, vitamins, and minerals. It can be served over rice, noodles, or enjoyed on its own for a wholesome and delicious plant-based option.

## Chickpea Curry

Chickpea Curry is a flavorful and satisfying dish made with chickpeas (also known as garbanzo beans) cooked in a spiced tomato-based sauce. The curry typically includes a variety of aromatic spices such as cumin, coriander, turmeric, and ginger, along with garlic, onions, and tomatoes. Additional ingredients like coconut milk or yogurt can be added for creaminess. Chickpea Curry offers a balance of protein, fiber, and rich flavors. It can be served with rice, naan bread, or roti for a complete and hearty meal. This vegetarian or vegan dish is loved for its warm and comforting qualities, making it a popular choice for Indian cuisine enthusiasts and curry lovers.

## Vegan Lentil Tacos

Vegan Lentil Tacos are a plant-based twist on the classic Mexican dish, replacing meat with hearty and protein-packed lentils. Cooked lentils are seasoned with a blend of spices like cumin, chili powder, and garlic powder to create a flavorful filling. The lentil mixture is then spooned into soft or crispy taco shells and topped with an array of fresh toppings such as diced tomatoes, lettuce, avocado, salsa, and vegan sour cream. Vegan Lentil Tacos offer a satisfying and delicious alternative for those following a vegan or vegetarian diet, while still providing the familiar and comforting flavors of traditional tacos. Enjoy these tasty and nutritious tacos as a fun and wholesome meal option.

## Roasted Vegetable Quinoa Salad

Roasted Vegetable Quinoa Salad is a wholesome and flavorful dish that combines roasted vegetables with protein-rich quinoa. A medley of colorful vegetables such as bell peppers, zucchini, eggplant, and cherry tomatoes are roasted until tender and slightly caramelized. Meanwhile, quinoa is cooked and fluffed to perfection. The roasted vegetables and quinoa are then tossed together with a tangy dressing made from ingredients like olive oil, lemon juice, and herbs. This salad offers a delightful combination of textures and flavors, with the sweetness of roasted vegetables complementing the nutty quinoa. It can be enjoyed as a satisfying main course or served as a side dish. This Roasted Vegetable Quinoa Salad is not only delicious but also packed with nutrients, making it a great choice for a nourishing and wholesome meal.

## Appetizer Recipes

### Stuffed Mushrooms

- Ingredients: Button mushrooms, breadcrumbs, minced garlic, chopped parsley, grated Parmesan cheese (or nutritional yeast for a vegan option), olive oil, salt, and pepper.
- Instructions: Remove the stems from the mushrooms and set them aside. In a bowl, mix breadcrumbs, minced garlic, chopped parsley, grated Parmesan cheese (or nutritional yeast), olive oil, salt, and pepper. Stuff the mushroom caps with the breadcrumb mixture and place them on a baking sheet. Bake in the oven at 375°F (190°C) for about 15-20 minutes or until the mushrooms are tender and the filling is golden brown.

### Vegan Spinach Artichoke Dip

- Ingredients: Frozen spinach, canned artichoke hearts, vegan cream cheese, vegan mayonnaise, nutritional yeast, minced garlic, onion powder, salt, and pepper.

- Instructions: Thaw and drain the frozen spinach and chop the artichoke hearts. In a mixing bowl, combine the spinach, artichoke hearts, vegan cream cheese, vegan mayonnaise, nutritional yeast, minced garlic, onion powder, salt, and pepper. Mix well until all ingredients are combined. Transfer the mixture to a baking dish and bake in the oven at 350°F (175°C) for about 20-25 minutes or until heated through and bubbly. Serve with bread, crackers, or vegetable sticks.

## Bruschetta

- Ingredients: Baguette or crusty bread, ripe tomatoes, fresh basil, minced garlic, extra virgin olive oil, balsamic vinegar, salt, and pepper.
- Instructions: Slice the baguette or bread into thick slices and toast them in the oven or on a grill until crispy. Meanwhile, dice the tomatoes and finely chop the fresh basil. In a bowl, mix the tomatoes, basil, minced garlic, olive oil, balsamic vinegar, salt, and pepper. Allow the flavors to meld for a few minutes. Once the bread slices are

toasted, spoon the tomato mixture onto each slice and serve.

## Veggie Spring Rolls

- Ingredients: Rice paper wrappers, thinly sliced vegetables (such as carrots, cucumbers, bell peppers), fresh herbs (such as cilantro, mint, basil), lettuce leaves, and a dipping sauce of your choice (such as peanut sauce or soy sauce).
- Instructions: Dip a rice paper wrapper in warm water for a few seconds until it becomes pliable. Place the wrapper on a clean surface and layer the thinly sliced vegetables, fresh herbs, and lettuce leaves in the center of the wrapper. Fold in the sides and roll up tightly, similar to a burrito. Repeat with the remaining ingredients. Serve the spring rolls with your preferred dipping sauce.

## Caprese Skewers

- Ingredients: Cherry tomatoes, fresh mozzarella balls, fresh basil leaves, balsamic glaze, skewers or toothpicks.

- Instructions: Skewer a cherry tomato, a fresh mozzarella ball, and a basil leaf onto each skewer or toothpick. Arrange the skewers on a serving platter and drizzle with balsamic glaze. Serve chilled.

These appetizer ideas offer a range of flavors and can be easily customized to suit your preferences. Enjoy creating these delicious bites for your next gathering or as a tasty snack.

## Deviled eggs

Deviled eggs are a classic appetizer made from hard-boiled eggs that have been cut in half and filled with a creamy mixture. The egg yolks are typically mixed with mayonnaise, mustard, and various seasonings like salt, pepper, and paprika. The filling is then spooned back into the egg white halves, creating a smooth and flavorful bite-sized treat. Deviled eggs are a popular party or picnic food, loved for their creamy texture, tangy flavor, and attractive presentation. They are a versatile dish that can be customized with different ingredients such as herbs, pickles, or even bacon, offering a variety of delicious options to suit individual tastes.

## strawberry Pineapple

Strawberry pineapple is a refreshing and vibrant combination of two delicious fruits. Strawberries are known for their sweet and juicy flavor, while pineapples offer a tropical and tangy taste. When combined, these fruits create a delightful balance of sweetness and acidity. Whether enjoyed on their own, in a fruit salad, or as an ingredient in various recipes, the pairing of strawberry and pineapple provides a burst of flavor and adds a tropical touch to any dish.

## Spicy Chicken Wing

Spicy chicken wings are a popular and flavorful appetizer or main dish. Chicken wings are typically seasoned with a combination of spices and sauces to give them a fiery kick. The wings are often marinated or coated in a spicy sauce made from ingredients such as hot sauce, chili powder, cayenne pepper, garlic, and other spices. They can be baked, grilled, or fried until crispy and golden brown. Spicy chicken wings are loved for their bold and zesty flavor, and they are often served with a side of blue cheese or ranch dressing for dipping. Whether enjoyed as a snack, party food, or part of a meal, spicy chicken wings are sure to satisfy those craving heat and deliciousness.

# Smoothies Recipes

## Strawberry Banana Smoothie

A traditional and delicious smoothie made with ripe bananas and luscious strawberries is the strawberry banana smoothie. This smoothie has a cool and creamy texture and is made with Greek yogurt, milk (dairy or plant-based), and, at your discretion, honey or maple syrup for sweetness. A pleasing flavor profile is produced by the natural creaminess of the bananas and the sweetness of the strawberries. The Strawberry Banana smoothie is a healthy and delectable option for breakfast, a snack, or a post-workout refreshment. It is packed with vitamins, fiber, and antioxidants. Enjoy this classic smoothie combination's fruity and creamy richness.

## Tropical Green Smoothie

Spinach, frozen mango chunks, pineapple, coconut milk, lime juice, and optional chia seeds are all combined to make the colorful and nutrient-dense Tropical Green smoothie. Combining the benefits of leafy greens with the sweetness of tropical fruits, this smoothie has a refreshing and tropical flavor. It gives you more energy and promotes general wellbeing because it is brimming with vitamins, minerals, and antioxidants. The Tropical Green Smoothie, when well blended, is a terrific way to increase your intake of greens while also indulging in the flavors of the tropics.

## Blueberry Avocado Smoothie

The vivid tastes of blueberries and the creamy consistency of ripe avocados are combined in a smoothie called blueberry avocado. This smoothie delivers a cooling and nutrient-rich beverage and is blended with spinach, almond milk, and the option of honey or agave syrup for sweetness. Antioxidants are provided by blueberries, and healthful fats and creaminess are added by avocado. A pleasantly well-balanced flavor is produced by the blending of the components. The blueberry avocado smoothie is a terrific way to start the day or have a nutritious snack because it is full of vitamins, minerals, and fiber. Enjoy this delightful and nourishing smoothie while you sip it.

## Peanut Butter Banana Smoothie

A creamy and filling beverage that blends the traditional tastes of peanut butter and banana is a peanut butter banana smoothie. This smoothie has a deep, nutty flavor and is made with ripe bananas, peanut butter, milk (dairy or plant-based), and can be optionally sweetened with honey or maple syrup. It's a fantastic source of potassium, good fats, and protein. The peanut butter and banana combine to make a delectably smooth texture when blended until smooth and creamy. Smoothies with peanut butter and bananas are a simple and wholesome breakfast or snack that gives you a surge of energy and a delicious flavor combination.

## Piña Colada Smoothie

Smoothies with the flavor profile of a pina colada are a tropical and revitalizing libation. These smoothies offer a lovely fusion of creamy and sweet flavors because they are made with frozen pineapple chunks, coconut milk, and occasionally Greek yogurt for extra creaminess. For an extra dash of tropical decadence, they can be personalized with alternative sweeteners like honey or agave syrup and topped with shredded coconut. When you want a taste of the tropics at any time of the day, pina colada smoothies are a terrific way to indulge in the tastes of pineapple and coconut in a healthier, non-alcoholic version.

## Desserts Recipes

1. Chocolate Avocado Mousse: A rich and creamy dessert made by blending ripe avocados, cocoa powder, sweetener of choice, and a splash of vanilla extract. The result is a decadent and healthier alternative to traditional chocolate mousse.

2. Vegan Banana Nice Cream: A simple and guilt-free dessert made by freezing ripe bananas and blending them until smooth and creamy. It can be enjoyed as is or customized with various flavors like peanut butter, cocoa powder, or mixed berries.

3. Fruit Parfait: A refreshing and colorful dessert consisting of layers of fresh or frozen fruits, yogurt or vegan coconut cream, and granola or nuts. It's a versatile dessert that allows for endless combinations of flavors and textures.

4. Chia Seed Pudding: A nutritious and easy-to-make dessert made by combining chia seeds with milk or plant-based milk, sweetener, and flavorings

like vanilla or cocoa powder. The mixture is left to thicken overnight, resulting in a creamy and pudding-like consistency.

5. Vegan Chocolate Chip Cookies: Classic chocolate chip cookies made without eggs or dairy. These cookies use plant-based substitutes like flax eggs, coconut oil, and dairy-free chocolate chips to create a delicious and vegan-friendly treat.

These are just a few examples of the many delightful vegan and plant-based desserts available. With a little creativity and the right ingredients, you can enjoy a wide variety of delicious and healthier sweet treats.

# Customized Recipe Templates

1. Recipe Template: Entrée

Title:

Ingredients:

- List all the ingredients with their quantities

Instructions:

1. Step-by-step instructions for preparing the dish
2. Number each step and provide clear details
3. Include cooking times and temperatures if necessary
4. Add any additional notes or tips for success

2. Recipe Template: Smoothie

Title:

Ingredients:

- List all the ingredients with their quantities

Instructions:

1. Step-by-step instructions for preparing the smoothie

2. Mention the order in which ingredients should be added to the blender
3. Include any optional add-ins or substitutions
4. Provide serving suggestions or garnishes if desired

3. Recipe Template: Baked Goods

Title:
Ingredients:
- List all the ingredients with their quantities

Instructions:
1. Step-by-step instructions for preparing the baked goods
2. Include details on mixing, kneading, or folding the dough/batter
3. Specify baking times and temperatures
4. Add any frosting or glazing instructions if applicable

Feel free to customize these templates based on your recipe requirements. Add or remove sections, include specific measurements, and provide detailed instructions to make your recipes clear and easy to follow. Happy cooking.

# Conclusion

The thyroid bolster recipe is designed to incorporate ingredients that are believed to support thyroid health. While it may offer some potential benefits, it's important to note that diet alone cannot cure or treat thyroid disorders. The recipe focuses on including foods rich in iodine, selenium, antioxidants, and other nutrients that are known to be beneficial for thyroid function.

However, it is crucial to approach the thyroid bolster recipe as a complementary component to a comprehensive treatment plan, including proper medical care, medication (if prescribed), and lifestyle modifications. Consulting with a healthcare professional or registered dietitian is essential to ensure that the recipe aligns with your specific needs and doesn't interfere with any existing conditions or medications.

Additionally, it's important to maintain a well-rounded, balanced diet that includes a variety of nutrient-dense foods. While certain ingredients in the thyroid bolster recipe may be beneficial, it's equally important to focus on overall nutritional intake and dietary diversity.

Remember, individual responses to dietary changes may vary, and it may take time to see any potential benefits. Monitoring your symptoms, working closely with your healthcare provider, and making informed choices based on your specific health needs are key to managing thyroid disorders effectively.

Disclaimer: The information provided here is for educational purposes only and should not be considered as medical advice. Always consult with a healthcare professional before making any significant changes to your diet or treatment plan.

# Recommendations

1. Consult a healthcare professional: If you have a thyroid disorder or suspect you may have one, it is important to seek medical advice and follow the recommended treatment plan. The thyroid bolster recipe can be used as a complementary approach alongside medical treatment, but it should not replace professional medical advice.

2. Incorporate thyroid-friendly foods: The recipe emphasizes foods such as sea vegetables (e.g., seaweed), Brazil nuts, berries, leafy greens, and omega-3 fatty acids (found in fatty fish and flaxseeds) that are considered beneficial for thyroid health. Include these foods in your diet regularly to support thyroid function.

3. Consider individual dietary needs: Everyone's dietary needs are unique, so it's important to tailor the recipe to your specific requirements. If you have any food allergies, sensitivities, or specific dietary restrictions, consult with a healthcare professional

or registered dietitian to make appropriate substitutions or modifications.

4. Maintain a balanced diet: The thyroid bolster recipe should be part of an overall balanced and nutritious diet. Ensure you're getting a variety of fruits, vegetables, whole grains, lean proteins, and healthy fats to support your overall health and well-being.

5. Lifestyle factors: In addition to diet, other lifestyle factors can impact thyroid health. Manage stress levels, prioritize sufficient sleep, engage in regular physical activity, and avoid smoking and excessive alcohol consumption.

Remember, while the thyroid bolster recipe may provide some potential benefits, it is not a substitute for medical treatment. Always consult with a healthcare professional for proper diagnosis, treatment, and guidance on managing your specific thyroid condition.

Printed in Great Britain
by Amazon

40982142R00050